Is appendectomy innocuous?

Or a possible function for the vermiform appendix

Constantin Panow

Copyright 2018

All rights reserved

Printed by Create Space

"Primum non nocere- First do no harm!"

Hippocrates (460-370BC)

Disclaimer

The author and publisher decline responsibility about any deleterious effect, which could result from wrong understanding, or interpretation and application of following text.

This publication is intended for information purposes only.

It can't replace consultations at a medical practitioner's office.

Key words

Appendicitis, appendectomy, bowel hormones, depressive syndrome, gastric tumors, weight loss, obesity, overweight, starches, carbohydrates, fibers, vegetables, fruit.

Contents

Copyright 2018 3

Disclaimer 6

Key words 7

Radiology 9

Tumors, inflammation 10

Measuring 12

Consequences 13

No carcinoids 15

Duodenal humoral response 16

Bewildering? 17

First incentive 17

Vegetables 19

Stomach tumors 20

My point 21

Modernity 24

Website 25

Radiology

Despite advances in modern imaging with ultrasound and scanner, appendectomy remains most frequently performed emergency surgical procedure.

Some data report a prevalence of more than 20% in industrialized countries.

With a mortality rate of 1.8%, medical doctors try to avoid this operation, even in our times of contemporaneity.

In disregard of this trend, few ask themselves about possible role of this organ in health and disease.

If 1976, when I started my studies in medicine, our teachers would admit that nothing is known about a possible function of appendix;

A lot of literature has been added in recent times.

Tumors, inflammation

We know for instance, that surgery at this target increases risk to have a colorectal carcinoma by 14%, and also of having Crohn's disease, but lowers incidence of ulcerative colitis.

We know since many years that the vermiform appendix is packed with Enterochromaffin cells (EC), and that serotonin activates substantially vagus nerve firing, thus promoting progression of stool and faster emptying of large bowel.

Constipation and nutrition habits play a serious role in prevalence of colon tumors.

Thus, at least this first relationship seems straightforward!

Perforation is the feared complication of this hollow and blind ending intestine.

It is due not to inflammation, but to obstruction in the outlet tract.

If previous data were unclear, now it is widely admitted that a large number of appendicitis cases resolve spontaneously.

In my experience this rate attains more than 80%. (Without rupture or abscess formation.)

Seasons

Prevalence of acute appendicitis is higher in summer months, probably owing to dehydration and harder stool formation.

In an older histological series pathologists noted degranulation of neuro-serotonin endings in inflamed but not obstructed organs.

This study was from a time when high incidence of spontaneously favorable course of this disease was ignored.

Now it is clear, that increased activity of these neurons promoted alleviation of plugging.

Measuring

In my practice as radiologist performing ultrasound, I observe acute appendicitis if transverse diameter is 1.5-1.8 cm (0.59-0.71 inches).

With dis-obstruction this cross section goes down rapidly to 0.8 cm (0.31 inches). Bowel wall remains though thick with more than 0.3 cm (0.12 inches).

This process takes several days to complete its full evolution to normal.

Consequences

Thus, from previous discussion it becomes clear that this part of our anatomy can in no way be insignificant to our health and general condition.

Serotonin is a small molecule, which crosses readily the blood-brain barrier.

It is produced in cells distributed in large bowel, but probably in biggest percentage mainly precisely in our vermiform appendix.

This minute compound is generated from amino acids, and especially directly from tryptophan.

Thus, ingestion of proteins keeps you longer with satiety sensation, as serotonin stimulates gratification and satisfaction centers in the central nervous system.

Ghrelin, also stimulated by serotonin attaches to growth-hormone releasing hormone receptor, which keeps up lipid and sugar content in blood.

Ghrelin, on the other hand drops as soon as the stomach is full, regardless of its content.

Ghrelin is known to be the main "hunger" hormone.

You remember the story of the conditioned reflex declared in Pavlov's dog model.

It is tightly linked to the parasympathetic system, while leptin stimulates the sympathetic one.

Both act on the same receptor in the brain, with opposite effects.

Ghrelin is produced mainly in the stomach, and the leptin-ghrelin chain is together responsible for activation of "satisfaction" centers in the central nervous system.

No carcinoids

Despite huge amount of serotonin cells in the appendix;

Localized masses of those encountered in some cases fail to demonstrate aggressive or malignant behavior known from carcinoids;

Which are tumors of similar Enterochromaffin cells in other body locations.

Duodenal humoral response

Lipids, proteins and sugars, starches ingested produce a large hormone response in proximal bowel.

Stomach emptying slows down, and stomach acid, lipase, trypsin and amylase production from pancreas increases tremendously.

Simple sugars and starches are rapidly transformed in glucose and stimulate insulin release from Langerhans' islet cells of pancreas. (So- called beta-cells).

Thus sugar in large quantities is driven inside all cells of the body.

Insulin production is counter-balanced by another minute peptide, which is called glucagon, and which in cases of hypo-glycaemia enhances gluconeogenesis and release of glucose from liver and muscle.

Both hormones are antagonized by somatostatin, another small peptide, which is produced in pancreas and small bowel.

Cholecystokinin secreted in duodenum empties gall-bladder and stimulates pancreatic exocrine secretion, with reverse down-regulation by this one.

It permits thus digestion of proteins and fat, and is very similar to gastrin, which stimulates stomach juice production.

Bewildering?

Now we need to implement all this rather baffling data in precise experimental models.

First scenario is composed of ingestion of all three macro-nutrients, proteins, lipids, and simple sugars and starches.

Then you arrive at the confusing framework, whose end-result is high-energy, high vitality system, with high expenditure.

Now, if burning of all this fuel becomes low, as in advancing age, or even in young adults with sedentary life-style, we have to do with increasing body weight.

Obesity ensues!

First incentive

Our main issue is to understand how this machinery works in order to avoid overweight.

Main actor has been pin-pointed in modern literature as being sugars.

Insulin drives them in huge quantities into cells, where they are transformed after a while of inactivity in fat.

Calorie restriction works for a while, but ends-up in a yo-yo phenomenon, rather unhealthy, and without desired effect, which would be weight loss on the long run.

One word here about fruit, which for most of them contain fructose.

This last compound does not activate significantly insulin secretion and is thus to be considered much healthier than simple sugars and starches.

On the contrary to old views that rice, bread, pasta and potatoes are complex sugars, this is no more tenable as a theory, but they are all four considered to be same as simple glucose.

If you are not convinced, check for glycemic index published widely in literature.

Unlike ancient perspective that the brain needs absolutely glucose for its function, this is also to be reviewed, as fuel can be provided from lipids in the liver, which transforms with fasting fat in ketone bodies.

In this situation we have to do with high ghrelin and growth hormone levels in blood circulation.

Vegetables

But the human body needs to be sustained with energy, and this one can be administered in the form of fiber carbohydrates, which are endowed with a much lower glycemic index.

This one is in vicinity of 0.1 for green salad, 0.2 for tomatoes and peppers, 0.3 for green and snap beans, lentils and green peas.

When such nutriments enter the stomach, this organ empties fast into duodenum, where secretion of digestion enzymes is low owing to somatostatin high levels and low output of all other gastro-intestinal peptides.

Thus breaking down of complex carbohydrates relies on intestinal flora and mucosal cell villi.

Forward transportation of bolus slows down.

As there is no compound which can ferment (as starches), bowel movement becomes ultra-slow.

Despite most articles claiming that cellulose, composed of D-glucose is indigestible by humans, I found evidence in literature pointing at the opposite. (Gut, 1984, 25, 805-810).

Probably D-glucose behaves with insulin like fructose does and provokes little excursion of this hormone.

Wide variation in our species exists in this regard.

As digestion of cellulose and absorption of D-glucose rely on other enzymes than pancreatic ones, these functions occur most probably by endocytosis of small bowel mucosal cells.

It is not excluded that even colon contributes to this process.

If there is danger of leakage of lectins through bowel wall cellular junctions with starch nutrition, this is most probably largely avoided with fiber-carbohydrate intake.

Those ones tamponade stomach acidity and as there is low level of all gastro-intestinal peptides (high somatostatin), gastrin is also suppressed.

Stomach tumors

It is important in this regard to absorb some fat in order to avoid the occurrence of a gastric cancer.

To be noted a very high level of this malignancy in vegetarian populations (Japan). I.e. a low-fat, low-protein diet.

Thus, if in a starch carbohydrate intake serotonin secreted by the vermiform appendix fosters rapid emptying of large bowel,

Not so with a fiber carbohydrate diet, in which serotonin would first promote increase of ghrelin-dependent Growth Hormone, and then only further effects on colon.

Recent literature suggests that high lipid consumption results in fat loss. (Provided essential fatty acids-Omega 3, 6, and 7 etc., cholesterol and phospholipids are included.)

Some protein intake is needed for amino-acid's renewal in this complex machinery.

My point

Thus, if you follow my reasoning, for above delineated purpose, only renouncement to simple sugars and starches is necessary.

With glucose and starch admission in one's diet, we observe high peaks of insulin, followed after a few hours by hypo-glycemic attacks.

Psychiatry

This is one factor explaining uneven mood in adepts of such "sweet regime".

Another reason is that most gastro-intestinal peptides cross readily the blood-brain barrier and boost effects on their own.

As for instance cholecystokinin is made responsible for panic and anxiety storms in the central nervous system.

Leptin and Ghrelin are tightly linked with centers of satisfaction;

While serotonin is known to have an anti-depressant effect.

Most medication for bipolar disorder nowadays relies on serotonin-like or serotonin reuptake inhibitor drugs.

You see how operating away this small blind ending loop of our bowel can have tremendous influence in our anatomy and function.

It would be easy to determine whether appendectomy is more prevalent between psychotic subjects.

Besides cholecystokinin plays probably a major role in patients with a gastro-duodenal ulcer, those ones being for most of them of an anxious personality.

Modernity

Changing life-style and nutrition habits is probably to be viewed as our future trend in therapy of disease and establishment of good health.

Besides, if it really occurs that the vermiform appendix should be preserved at operation, then probably you would find some surgeons happy to operate you twice. Or several times?

Perpetuating the target organ is certainly another tendency in modern medicine.

Website

I hope you enjoyed this short text.

You can reach me at

www.thenopillshealthprospect.com

If you have any questions or comments, don't hesitate, write in my blog!

www.ingramcontent.com/pod-product-compliance
Lightning Source LLC
Chambersburg PA
CBHW030042230526
45472CB00002B/629